DEMENTIA PSYCHOLOGY

CONNOR WHITELEY

No part of this book may be reproduced in any form or by any electronic or mechanical means. Including information storage, and retrieval systems, without written permission from the author except for the use of brief quotations in a book review.

This book is NOT legal, professional, medical, financial or any type of official advice.

Any questions about the book, rights licensing, or to contact the author, please email connorwhiteley@connorwhiteley.net

Copyright © 2023 CONNOR WHITELEY

All rights reserved.

DEDICATION
Thank you to all my readers without you I couldn't do what I love.

INTRODUCTION

Dementia is not a pleasant disease or condition in the slightest and I personally wouldn't wish in on my worst enemy.

Personally, like so many families, I lost an amazing Great-Uncle to dementia in 2021 after years of watching him deteriorate, my family suffer the emotional pain or watching him basically die and it was a horrible time for everyone.

Since that time, my family has slowly recovered from the death of such a great person, but the memory of all those awful years continues.

As well as since I am a psychology student, author and podcast, this meant I was in a very fortunate position because of amazing readers like you to research and actually do anything constructive with the grief caused by the death.

Therefore, I wanted to write this engaging easy-to-understand book to learn for myself, my audience and others what is dementia, how to prevent dementia and so many other great facets of this fascinating topic.

Whilst this introduction might seem like this book came out of sadness about a death (which it did in a way), it really came from a burning curiosity to find out more about dementia and most importantly, help raise awareness of this awful condition.

What Will This Book Cover?

This great easy-to-understand book covers a lot of great facets of dementia science that covers cognitive psychology, biological psychology, neuropsychology and many more.

We start off by looking at the interesting topic of what is dementia and the different types. That will definitely surprise you because there is a lot more than you realised (I know there was for me).

Then we move onto the different ways to prevent dementia and that is absolutely critical to the purpose of this book, and it is such an great read since most of the tips are so easy to implement.

All before we move onto the final section of the book that investigates brilliant facets of dementia science that you never would have considered before. Like the possibility of dementia rates actually declining, sleep disorder and more. Before we finish off the book by looking at the fascinating topic of inequalities in dementia healthcare.

That is a real eye-opener.

Who Is This Book For?

As always my books are definitely not written like boring dull textbooks that we all know and love from our university days. I always try and keep my books engaging, conversational and like a friend is telling you the information.

Also like the rest of my books, they're written for psychology students, psychology professionals and anyone that is interested in psychology.

And whilst none of the information in this book is any sort of official advice, if you're looking for a fun, engaging book on dementia science then definitely look no further.

Who Am I?

Personally I always love to know who the author is of the nonfiction I write so I know for sure that the information is coming from a good source. In case you're like me, I'm Connor Whiteley, the author of over 30 psychology books and I'm the host of the weekly The Psychology World Podcast available on all major podcast apps and YouTube, where each week we look at another psychology topic and the latest psychology news.

Additionally, I am a psychology student at the University of Kent, England studying a specialised clinical psychology degree. As well as this book has plenty of references and citations at the end of the book so you know that all the information is backed up by science and research.

Now that we know more about each other, let's

dive in and start learning about the great world of dementia.

PART ONE: WHAT IS DEMENTIA?

WHAT IS DEMENTIA AND TYPES OF DEMENTIA?

To kick off our dementia journey, I wanted us to first look at this blog post I wrote last year for an episode of The Psychology World Podcast that serves as a great introduction to this topic.

It covers what is dementia and the wide range of types of dementia, including some you have probably never ever heard of (I know I hadn't).

Enjoy.

***

<u>What Is Dementia and Types of Dementia?</u>

After experiencing a personal loss to dementia in early 2021, I really want to raise awareness about Dementia and some ways to keep our brains healthy. This is extremely important considering that research shows up to 40% of Dementia cases are preventable. Also I'm mentioning this on a psychology podcast because Dementia causes severe cognitive decline in people, so it's of interest to us from a cognitive psychology and clinical psychology viewpoint.

What Is Dementia?

Dementia isn't a single thing.

Instead, it's an umbrella term for a wide range of conditions that we'll look at later. This is similar to the umbrella term we all know, Anxiety as anxiety can be broken down into Phobias, Generalised Anxiety Disorder, Social Anxiety Disorder and more.

Furthermore, dementia impacts a lot of functions like speech, thinking patterns and memory. As well as in terms of the neurological damage, dementia attacks the brain and eventually kills the brain cells of a person.

Interestingly enough, this can leave the brain around 140 grams lighter than a healthy brain.

Personally, as much as I want to draw on my own experience, I'm not comfortable sharing that so openly. But I do want to say how scary this condition is because you basically watch one of your loved ones slipping away until they only become a shell for someone (who isn't your loved one) to be there.

Dementia isn't a condition that we should leave because it only affects the older people in society because it can affect people in their early 50s too.

Causes and Types of Dementia:

As the main audience for this podcast are psychology students and psychology professionals, I guess this should come as no surprise that dementia does not have one cause, it has many. Since it can be caused by a number of brain diseases and whilst

Alzheimer's is the most common disease, it is far from the only one. And each one has its own early warning signs to watch out for.

Therefore, for the rest of the podcast episode, you're going to hear about some of the types of dementia and what their early warning signs are.

Alzheimer's Disease

With this being the most common dementia disease with 50% to 75% of dementia suffers having this condition, dementia scientists know a lot about it. Meaning we know Alzheimer's develops due to a strange build-up of proteins in certain parts of the brain. For example, the brain areas that are responsible for memory and spatial navigation. Then over time this strange build up spreads to other areas of the brain. Leading to the sufferer developing more severe symptoms.

In terms of early warning signs, here are some:

- Getting lost
- Getting confused by the time of day or the date
- Regularly forgetting names, events and faces

And it's that *regularly* that is important because we all forget names, faces and events from time to time, it's normal. But it's when it happens regularly that we should at least be warn something could be wrong.

Vascular Dementia

This is another one that I hear about quite often and this occurs when blood flow is reduced to the brain, meaning the brain cells don't are enough oxygen and nutrients. Leading to the brain cells to die.

It's this damage that is called Vascular dementia.

However, one of the problems with this condition is because the reduction of blood can happen to any part of the brain, it can affect everyone in different ways.

This only adds to problems for researchers because you cannot treat people with this condition as a uniform group in your samples. And as psychology people, I know we all face struggles with this problem. For example, just because you use university psychology students in your study, it doesn't mean you can treat them all the same. Especially when you start to consider their cultural experiences, attitudes, sexualities, genders and more.

Yet some warning signs are:

- Changes in personality
- Slower thinking
- Disorientation and difficulty walking

Dementia with Lewy Bodies

Moving onto our penultimate type of dementia, this is where things start to get really interesting because we're now talking about the types I've never heard of before.

Therefore, Lewy Bodies are small chunks of protein that develop inside the nerve cells in the parts of the brain responsible for thinking, movement and memory. As a result, Lewy Bodies disrupt the nerve signals in the cells and over time they cause the nerve cells to die.

The warning signs are:
- Visual hallucinations and vivid dreams
- Changes in alertness and confusion
- Stiffness, trembling and difficulty walking

Frontotemporal Dementia

Personally I think this is a very scary form of dementia to think about because… well I'll just tell you about it.

Unlike other forms of dementia, this disease doesn't attack cells pre se. Instead it makes the front part of the brain smaller, which as we know from Biological Psychology is responsible for our emotions, personality, higher-order reasoning and more.

All in all this is the part of the brain that makes us, us.

Meaning when this part of the brain shrinks and proteins build up in this area, it causes a person's personality to change in a number of ways.

Here are the early warning signs:
- Changes in diet or overeating
- Lack of personal awareness
- Lack of understanding, empathy or social awareness

Conclusion

Overall there are a lot of different types of dementia but I hope after reading or listening to this podcast episode, you have a better understanding of dementia. It's a horrible, awful disease but like everything if we keep researching it and becoming more aware of it. Then hopefully we can do something about dementia in the future.

We've already come a long way in our understanding, but we are nowhere near done so I hope if anything, this podcast has given you a bit more awareness about this awful, brutal disease.

WHY DEMENTIA ISN'T A DIAGNOSIS?

Now that we know what dementia actually is as well as what some of the different types of dementia are, I wanted us to look at another blog post I wrote recently about a very interesting concept. Since dementia itself isn't a diagnosis, and this flies in the face of a lot of medical doctors and other professionals.

But this is a brand new way of thinking that could have very powerful impacts and it is a brilliant concept to learn about.

You'll enjoy this next chapter.

***

<u>Why Dementia Isn't A Diagnosis?</u>

Continuing our clinical psychology look at dementia, I want to talk about this fascinating topic that no one thinks about. I certainly didn't. It's the topic of dementia isn't a diagnosis and if we stop there, then the dementia sufferer cannot get the professional help they need. And what makes this really interesting is how this relates to other areas of psychology too. You don't want to miss this!

<u>Why Dementia Isn't A Diagnosis?</u>

On past dementia-focused podcast episodes, we've spoken about the different types of dementia and how they all differ. Each one has its own causes, symptoms and possible treatment options to some extent. As well as dementia is just an umbrella term for a whole range of mental health conditions.

Therefore, if anyone just says someone has dementia then this can be extremely dangerous. As it can stop them from getting professional help and seeking a real diagnosis to find out what condition they have exactly.

This is even more important when we realise that several conditions copy the symptoms of dementia and have similar impacts on behaviour. Hence why this is of interest to psychology.

Furthermore, not only does it allow people to understand the type of dementia they have. But it allows us all to understand what aspects of our cognition and behaviour are likely to be affected first and those likely to be affected later.

So by getting a specific diagnosis, it allows us to plan more effectively with treatment and support, but expectations too.

Another way to think about this is like saying someone has a headache. Due to headaches can be caused by an entire range of things, like stress and migraines. As well as they can be caused by a range of diseases which can be much more serious, like brain tumours and strokes.

This is why it is critical to always get a professional diagnosis.

Additionally, if we apply this to clinical psychology more generally, this is why diagnosis is important for all mental health conditions. For example, people could believe a child is awful, badly behaved and anti-social but they might have autism. And without the diagnosis we wouldn't know and we wouldn't know how to get access to the brilliant range of support and interventions that could be used to help the child cope with everyday life and thrive.

Importance of Checking and Reversible Causes of Dementia:

Another reason to check for dementia and get a real diagnosis is because it is critical to check for reversible causes of dementia. This is another great reason why I love learning about dementia because I had no idea dementia had reversible causes, meaning the dementia can be reversed.

Some reversible causes of dementia include:

- A B12 deficiency
- Hypothyroidism
- Chronic infection like in Lyme disease.

All these conditions and causes can be easily detected by blood tests so after a diagnosis has been reached, these tests can be conducted and hopefully if the causes are reversible. Then a treatment programme can be arranged and the dementia can be gone.

In addition, we'll look at this potentially reversible cause of dementia in another episode, but depression is another cause to bear in mind.

Also by using structural brain imaging, doctors can identify subdural hematomas (accumulation of blood between the skull and the brain) and other rather horrific sounding abnormalities that need to be removed to relieve brain pressure or help prevent strokes.

Overall, it's important to get a real dementia diagnosis so people can understand the type of dementia they have so treatment options can be developed. Even if it is sadly just options to slow down the dementia. As well as it gives people a chance to see if their dementia is reversible. (I really wish my Great-uncle had that option)

More On Treatment For Dementia:

Throughout the podcast episode, I've hinted (heavily!) at the main reason why getting the right diagnosis is important for treatment options. Since it is only with the right diagnosis can the sufferer get the correct treatment for them.

For example:

- Cholinesterase inhibitors can improve patients with Alzheimer's, dementia with Lewy bodies and vascular dementia.
- Stroke Workup and treatment is necessary for vascular dementia and it usually uses aspirin or other blood thinners.

- Surgical Evaluation and possible intervention is needed for people with normal pressure hydrocephalus (a build-up of spinal fluid inside the brain) or subdural hematoma.
- Selective Serotonin Reuptake Inhibitors (very famous in clinical psychology!) are used as the first line of defence (and first therapy) for treating frontotemporal dementia.

Then of course, don't forget about medical trials or studies looking at new treatments of dementia. None of this is official advice, but there are some great studies going on for dementia, my placement supervisor is always working on one (I think). Therefore, if you and the dementia sufferer are interested in that sort of stuff, go for it! Explore the area and you never ever know you might have helped dementia science take another step forward!

Why Does This Apply To Psychology Students and Professionals? Conclusion:

I know this podcast is made up mainly of amazing psychology students and psychology professionals and this is for whom I always try to create my content for. But I wouldn't blame you in the slightest for wondering why I'm telling you about the importance of diagnosis, since it is a fundamental principle in clinical psychology.

But I did this episode for two main reasons. Reasons that might not be clear to us, but they are critical for our clients and the people we serve.

Firstly, don't give our clients a general diagnosis

like dementia. Because at the end of the day, that general diagnosis is useless to them, give them the full details so they can truly understand what is happening to them, and maybe they can start to do something about it.

Of course, this doesn't always apply, but you get the idea. As well as it will help them to understand why psychotherapy or another course of action is needed.

Secondly, deepen our understanding. I still love clinical psychology because there is always something more to learn, and for all of us deepening our understanding and learning about where people are coming from is critical.

By learning why dementia isn't a good diagnosis, we can inform our own practices and learn how to treat our current or future clients better. And learning more about clinical psychology never hurts, does it?

Overall, dementia is a great topic that has as many facets as other mental health conditions, so it is important to focus on from time to time. But remember the most important takeaway from this episode is don't settle for a *dementia* diagnosis.

WHAT IS VASCULAR DEMENTIA?

I know we sort of looked at this type of dementia in the last chapter but I really want to zoom in on it, because it is actually rather interesting.

Therefore, vascular dementia is caused by strokes, but it actually isn't as simple as that. Since you have vascular cognitive impairment as well. These are mildly cognitive impairments that are caused by strokes.

As well as the problem with the word *stroke* is that it's used so much but no one ever defines it when they're talking about it, or they don't explain what it involves. Since the only accurate comparison I've heard until now is that a stroke is like a fire in the brain.

That's a great comparison in a non-clinical context because it helps people to understand how destructive and serious it is.

However, as this is a psychology book, we need to be a bit more detailed than that. Therefore, strokes happen in a person when an artery sending blood from the heart to the brain is blocked off. Then this part of the brain doesn't receive enough blood (which contains the all-important oxygen) and dies.

As a result of the problem being associated to blood vessels, strokes are rightly (in my opinion) called "vascular disease" or sometimes "cerebrovascular disease" to emphasis the problem is with blood vessels in the brain or cerebrum.

Moving a bit closer towards dementia, other people and family members normally notice a major stroke in their loved one when large arteries are blocked straight away. Due to the effects are so clear and stark and worrying.

However, tiny strokes from when small and microscopic arteries in the brain experiencing blockages are typically silent. And it is only when lots of these are blocked or have had smaller strokes does this cause problems with memory and thinking, with these tiny strokes normally being accidentally discovered on a brain scan or CT scan.

In addition, it is almost normal for most people to have had a handful of these little strokes by the time they reach their 70s and 80s. Along with these tiny strokes are generally too small to cause dementia by themselves (thankfully), but they can make thinking and memory worse in people who have another condition as well. For example Alzheimer's disease.

Moreover, when strokes are the primary cause of

thinking and memory problems, this is when we use the term "vascular dementia" if a person's daily functioning is impaired and "vascular cognitive impairment" if their daily function is normal.

Now we know that strokes are very bad for us, our cognition and our risk of getting dementia. What are the main risk factors?

<u>Major Risk Factors For Strokes:</u>

Some of the medical risk factors for strokes including:

- Prior stroke
- Heart disease
- Prior stroke warning sign. Like transient ischemic attack or TIA
- Diabetes
- High blood pressure
- High cholesterol
- A disease of other blood vessels of the body

Nonetheless, medical factors aren't the only things that can increase your chance of having a stroke, because your lifestyle can increase your risk too.

- Obesity
- Unhealthy diet
- More than one drink of alcohol a day
- Smoking
- Sedentary lifestyle

Whilst I'm sure a lot of you probably laughed or gasped at the "More than one drink of alcohol a day" one (and I know plenty of my friends would agree with you), it just goes to show how many different factors can increase your chance of having a stroke, and in the context of this book, dementia too.

Although, thankfully all of these factors can be controlled and healthier habits can be adopted to lower these risk factors to decrease your overall risk of having a stroke. Allowing you to live a healthier life.

I must admit though that there are some factors that cannot be changed whatsoever unfortunately. For example, the risk that when a person is over the age of 55, their risk of a stroke doubles every decade.

That's why it's important to try to make your risk of having a stroke low in the first place, so that doubling effect isn't doubling too dramatically, if you catch my drift.

And of course, whilst none of this book is ever any sort of official advice, talking to your doctor, researching healthy eating and more are all great techniques to hopefully decrease your overall risk. Your doctor is definitely a great place to start as they're not only the experts in the medical field, but they know *your* body and how to help *you*.

PART TWO: REDUCING YOUR RISK OF DEMENTIA

DEMENTIA PSYCHOLOGY

5 WAYS TO KEEP YOUR BRAIN HEALTHY AND REDUCE YOUR RISK OF DEMENTIA

Moving onto the next section of the book that focuses on preventing dementia, which is something we sort of preluded to in the last section, there are plenty of great tips and tricks that are very easy to do to help prevent dementia.

Therefore, over the next two chapters, we're going to explore ten different ways to help you reduce your risk of getting dementia. Starting off with this blog post I did for the podcast back in 2021 before I even knew that I wanted to do more episodes on the topic, and I wanted to write a book too.

Enjoy.

***

Continuing with our look at dementia, which will be a focus in 2022, I wanted to share with you some ways to reduce your risk of getting dementia and keeping your brain healthy. And whilst people tend to think about these methods later in life, it's important to think about keeping your brain healthy in any part of life.

As well as Dementia Experts say that keeping your brain healthy in your forties and fifties is critical when it comes to preventing dementia. But whenever you decide to make changes to keep your brain healthy, you would see a great overall benefit to your health!

Ways To Keep Your Brain Healthy:

Avoid Smoking:

We've all heard the different ways that smoking damages your physical health and it links to a number of different medical conditions. But in terms of your mind and mental health, studies have shown that smoking increases your risk of developing diseases like Alzheimer's and Vascular Dementia.

In addition, as psychology students and professionals, we all know the psychology of addiction and why it is hard to give up smoking. But maybe thinking about it as a way to protect your brain, reduce your risk and preserve your cognitive abilities for the long term, might just give you or your loved ones the motivation to stop.

As well as there are plenty of professional websites to find tips to help you stop smoking on the internet.

Staying Connected

This definitely links into [How 100 Year Olds Keep Their Minds Sharp?](#) but as we're talking about dementia it is very important to stay connected with people regardless of our age.

As staying connected means we still have to

absorb lots of social stimuli that keeps our minds sharp, engaged and active. This all contributes to keeping our brains healthy, and this is why it's a good idea to join clubs, go to senior centres and be active in older age as it keeps them connected to wider society.

Additionally, more and more research is suggesting that enjoyable face to face interactions can slow the symptoms of dementia. For example, deteriorating memory as listening and responding to people requires quick thinking and responding.

Keeping Your Blood Pressure and Cholesterol In Check

Something I'm starting to notice is how many different areas of psychology dementia fits into as it touches on clinical psychology, cognitive psychology, biological psychology and more.

And that's what's interesting about dementia.

Anyway, having high blood pressure and high cholesterol can cause you to experience a lot of different health problems, so it's important to keep them in check. As well as keeping them in check does reduce your risk of developing dementia.

Consequently, if you wanted to reduce your cholesterol, you could reduce your consumption of biscuits, cheese and red meats and increase the amount of fruit, vegetables and oily fish that you eat.

Eating Well and Balanced

Now I'm definitely going to define what this actually means because we have all heard this so many times, but no one ever tells us what a balanced diet and eating well means.

Therefore, eating well and balanced is a great way to reduce your risk of developing several health conditions in later life. And what it means is eating a balanced diet could help to reduce your risk of dementia by reducing your risk of cardiovascular disease.

In addition, eating well means eating healthy. But it doesn't mean cutting fats out altogether as some fats like those found in oily fish, nuts, seeds and avocado do have health benefits. As well as a good balance of fibre, fruits, vegetables every week can go a long way to keeping your body healthy and giving it the nourishment it needs.

And in case I'm losing anyone because this is a psychology podcast and they don't see a psychology connection. The connection is by keeping your brain healthy (the brain is covered by cognitive, biological and neuropsychology too), it reduces your risk of developing various conditions that can cause your cognitive abilities to decline, which results in your behaviour changing. As well as human behaviour is the purpose of psychology so that's the connection in case you were a bit lost.

Exercise And Keep Your Brain Active:

Whilst this has been mentioned on the last Brain health episode, I want to remind you of it because keeping your brain both mentally and socially active is vital to reduce your risk of dementia. As it keeps your brain busy and processing information. This can be as simple as learning, doing puzzles, crosswords, listening to a certain psychology podcast (Ha!) or reading nonfiction books.

It's all about keeping your brain active and making sure it has new information to process. That's the real key.

5 OTHER WAYS TO REDUCE DEMENTIA RISK

Continuing on from the last chapter, we're now going to be looking at another five ways to reduce your risk of dementia. And I know that some of these seem too easy, common sense and more, but as I mentioned a few chapters ago, that's half the problem.

As a result of how easy they are, people just don't do them and they don't try to modify their lifestyle and habits to incorporate some of these tips into them, and that might actually increase their risk of dementia overtime.

***

In this is clinical psychology episode of The Psychology World Podcast, we've going to be talking about 5 Ways to Keep Your Brain Healthy and Reduce the Risk of Getting Dementia.

Personally, I really wanted to do this episode because we have a dementia suffer in our family. And

I really don't want any of you to go through this so hopefully this could help you, your family and your clients.

5 Ways to Keep Your Brain Healthy and Reduce the Risk of Getting Dementia

Get your Flu vaccination:

Surprisingly enough, becoming vaccinated against the flu has other benefits because it may help to protect you against Alzheimer's disease. Since psychology research studied a large data set of 9066 people and they found people who got a flu vaccination had a decreased risk of cognitive decline. This is associated with Alzheimer's.

Additionally, the researchers added: "…people that consistently got their annual flu shot had a lower risk of Alzheimer's. This translated to an almost 6% reduced risk of Alzheimer's disease for patients between the ages of 75-84 for 16 years."

Personally, I think this is a great point because it shows by protecting our physical health, we can protect our mental health too. Also, it's reasonably easy to do.

Be Positive:

I have said this before so please check out the other clinical psychology podcast episodes for more information. But being a positive, cheerful person is always great. And thankfully, positivism isn't an innate trait so it can be learnt if you're not positive at the moment.

If you want to start becoming more positive, then maybe start my appreciating the small things.

Like, thanking your loved ones, being grateful for your health and maybe write about why something positive each day.

Get a good night sleep:

I think this is a certainly interesting point because we all know we need to get enough sleep and I talk about this a lot more in Biological Psychology.

However, whilst researchers are still trying to determine the relationship between Dementia and sleep. Some research clearly shows the brain gets rid of a lot of its waste during sleep that is associated with Alzheimer's disease.

Meaning if you get more sleep then you're less likely to get Dementia.

Add berries, apples and green tea to your diet:

Moving onto some more diet-based ways to keep your brain healthy. Research has shown people should eat foods high in flavonoids, substances that reduce inflammation, and these types of foods are associated with a reduction in Dementia.

Therefore, eating berries, apples and drinking green tea can be protective factors to keep your brain healthy and dark chocolate is high in flavonoids too.

Personally, I'm grateful for this fact because I really eat a lot of fruit and sometimes I drink green tea. So, hopefully, I'm on the right track.

Drink Coffee

However, if you don't like the taste of green tea and I can understand why. I hated it at first! It turns out by drinking coffee it has dementia reducing effects in addition to its increase in short term concentration.

According to a longitudinal study of 1409 people, people who drunk moderate amounts of coffee a day, 3 to 5 cups, in mid-life reduce the risk of Alzheimer's disease later in life.

This is another point I'm happy about because I tend to drink two to three cups a day.

Nonetheless, I did want to mention maybe two years ago, I read a study linking drinking over four cups of coffee a day with increase mortality later in life. Of course, it was years ago and I don't have a reference for it. But whilst we're on the topic of being healthy, I thought I should give a caveat.

PART THREE: ADDITIONAL INFORMATION ABOUT DEMENTIA

DEMENTIA PSYCHOLOGY

DEMENTIA AND SLEEPING DISORDER

To open the final section of the book focusing on other interesting findings to do with dementia, I wanted to open with a look at sleeping disorders. Since I was rather surprised to final out that they were actually rather common, so there's a link between sleeping disorders and dementia.

And as this is book looking at dementia, it is something we just have to look at in more fascinating depth.

As a result, it turns out between 40% to 60% of patients with dementia are affected by insomnia, up to 25% of patients with some form of mild dementia has some kind of sleep disorder and this increases to 50% of dementia patients with moderate to severe cases of dementia.

This is interesting to look at because this isn't something we tend to hear about when it comes to dementia for a range of reasons, so this is definitely going to be an eye-opening chapter for sure.

Additionally, a literature review by Da Silva (2015) found that sleep disturbances frequently occur in patients with dementia as well as this was a predictor of cognitive decline in older people with dementia.

Therefore, the review suggested it was possible that by identifying and treating sleep disorders in people with dementia and with mild cognitive impairment, this may help preserve their cognition, and monitoring these sleep disturbances in patients with mild cognitive impairment might help identify the initial symptoms of dementia.

In terms of dementia, the primary sleep problems that patients with all forms of dementia experience are insomnia, excessive daytime sleepiness, altered circadian rhythms, and excessive movement during the night. For instance, leg kicks, acting out dreams, and wandering.

Also one of the most serious sleep problems is the circadian linked phenomenon of "sundowning" were people in the evening hours regularly begin to have a delirium-like state with confusion, anxiety, agitation, and aggressive behaviour with potential for wandering away from home.

And another reason why this is critical to study is because sleeping difficulties in dementia patients is often a reason for becoming early institutionalised, and this wandering results in the need for patients to stay in locked units.

In fact, I know haven't done this a lot in the book but I wanted to mention something that happened to my Great-Uncle with dementia. Since he used to wake up in the middle of the night and act like it was the start of the day with him having a shave (something that was almost dangerous at this stage with the dementia) so by wonderful Great-Aunt had to get up to, help him and convince him to go back to bed despite his protests that it was the start of the day.

She did that every night for about probably 5 years. I admire her commitment but I really understand why some family members place them in a care home.

At the end of the day, if you have someone who is affected by dementia, you need to do what's right for them AND yourself to. If you're going to be burnout and your mental health destroyed by looking after them, there is absolutely NO shame in putting them in a care facility.

And I can say that because me and my family have lived it.

The Difference Between *Normal* Sleeping Problems and Dementia

As most of the readers here have studied psychology and have a pretty good basic knowledge of human behaviour, I wanted to jump in here in case you're thinking this is a lot of fuss over sleeping problems when it is normal at this later age in life.

Personally, I completely agree up to a point so I

wanted to make it clear with research why it is critical to understand the difference between normal and dementia-related sleeping problems.

Since Cassidy-Eagle & Siebern (2017) found that nearly 40% of people aged over 65 reported some form of sleeping disorder and 70% of people over 65 have four or more co-morbid illnesses.

So that's suggests that sleeping disorders and problems at this age are rather common.

This is even more supported by the fact that as people age sleep gets more fragmented and deep sleep declines (Biological Psychology). As well as people get less active and healthy with this contributing to an increase in problems like insomnia.

However, as we've seen in the previous chapters, not getting a good night sleep is bad for risk of getting dementia. Due to changes occur more frequently as well as severely in people with mild cognitive impairments. So spending more time awake in bed and taking longer to fall asleep have been associated with increased risk of developing dementia or mild cognitive decline in older adults.

Overall, whilst yes it is almost common for older adults to have sleeping problems, it is equally important that they get sorted out so the risk of dementia hopefully remains the same or lower for that person. And that's all before we consider the sleeping problems for people with dementia like the story about my Great-Uncle.

How Do We Treat These Problems?

Thankfully there are some great ways to treat these sleeping problems in older adults and dementia sufferers. For instance Cognitive Behavioural Therapy (CBT) is effective at treating insomnia in both older and younger adults. Also older adults find CBT more acceptable than medication treatment because it has no side effects associated with the drugs for insomnia.

Another study supporting CBT is Cassidy-Eagle & Siebern (2017) who used CBT to treat 28 older adults with insomnia and mild cognitive impairment. The results showed improved sleep and improved measurements of executive functioning like planning and memory. This indicates that CBT could be a helpful intervention for patients suffering with mild cognitive impairment.

Then again, more research does need to be done to fully explore the potential benefits, but at least the signs are very positive.

In addition, casting our minds back to the beginning of the chapter about the primary sleeping problems dementia patients face. The first step to help treat the problems is the doctors need to identify any other sleep or medical conditions so they can be treated. Resulting in the reduction of insomnia and excessive daytime sleepiness.

This is about taking a holistic approach which I am always a fan of, because it's all well and good kicking the insomnia, for example, but if the patient still has other problems that will affect their sleep. Then treating the insomnia was almost pointless in a way.

Bright light therapy is another great therapy here because it can keep a person more alert during the day, and when combined with melatonin, it can help regularise the person's circadian rhythm.

Finally, behavioural habits can be powerful here too for treatment. For example, limiting your caffeine intake before you go to bed, going for a long walk outside in the early morning so your body knows it's the start of the day, and the same when it gets dark so your body knows it's getting near the end of the day and your body needs to start preparing itself to go to sleep, amongst other behavioural things you can do.

Overall, I'm still surprised there's a lot to sleeping problems, conditions and dementia but that's the amazing thing about dementia and the human body. There are so many interconnected aspects that we need to focus on.

And that's why this is a great topic to learn about because you never know when you'll come across something surprising.

HOW CAN DEMENTIA RELATE TO CRIMINAL BEHAVIOUR?

Personally I completely agree with you if you're thinking that dementia couldn't possibly have an impact on criminal behaviour. When I first came across the research that I turned into a podcast episode, I was rather shocked by it all because it was just so surprising.

However, I really wanted to include it in the book to highlight how important tackling dementia is, because it has a lot of wide ranging impacts and negative outcomes that lots of people don't think about.

Including the impacts mentioned in this great next chapter.

Enjoy.

***

Continuing with our fascinating look at dementia, we're going to move away from clinical psychology and into forensic psychology to see how dementia can impact criminal behaviour. This will be a perfect episode for anyone who loves forensic and criminal psychology!

How Can Dementia Impact Criminal Behaviour?

As a society as a whole, we are never too surprised when a criminal that has committed crimes before gets in trouble. But when a 60 year old model citizen commits a crime even if it is only vaguely illegal, we become a lot more shocked and we really want to know what happened.

And it turns out dementia can be one such explanation.

Since Liljegren et al. (2015) conducted a study that suggests that new late-onset criminal behaviour could reflect an underlying dementia. And as we've mentioned before, dementia is an umbrella term for a wide range of conditions.

Also, rather interestingly, the different crimes committed actually differ with each type of dementia.

This particular study involved a retrospective record review of patients that were seen at the University of California between 1999 and 2013. That revealed that out of the 545 people with Alzheimer's Disease examined only 8% of them got into any legal trouble, and they only tended to get into legal trouble when the dementia symptoms were well established.

For example, people with dementia could drive the wrong way on a motorway or they could wander onto private property, also known as trespassing. Due to they're confused. As well as dementia sufferers could walk out of a store without realising they hadn't paid for such an item.

Therefore, these "crimes" are very understandable when we find out the person has dementia.

On the other hand, there are other criminal behaviours that don't occur in Alzheimer's patients. For example, socially inappropriate actions (like sexual harassment), fighting and public urination. These types of behaviours are common in another type of dementia we haven't looked at yet, called behavioural variant Frontotemporal Dementia (bvFTD).

Furthermore, Liljegren et al. (2015) reported that out of the 171 with bvFTD they examined 37% of them got into legal trouble with these socially inappropriate behaviours.

What Is Behavioural Variant Frontotemporal Dementia?

This type of dementia tends to occur in people when they're in their 50s and it is characterised as a gradual onset of personality changes including inappropriate and impulsive behaviours.

In addition, over time these behaviours become more and more pronounced and clear to see. Then the cognitive changes with this type of dementia include memory, organisational skills and language do actually develop and start to return. Yet this is only after the behavioural changes.

However, the early brain damage in behavioural

variant Frontotemporal Dementia occurs in the brain regions that are a part of the brain's "emotional salience network". And this is a critical network because involves regions such as the amygdala and the insular cortex. Both of these areas are known for their importance in emotional regulation.

An Important Wider Forensic Psychology Point:

Nonetheless, there is a critical point to all of this criminal behaviour and mental health condition talk. There are other conditions like bipolar disorder, sociopathy and alcohol abuse that can also lead to criminal behaviour.

Therefore, when people are arrested and it is believed they might have a mental health condition that impacted their criminality. It is important for them to get assessed by a health care professional so we can fully understand what happened.

As well as this is why different disciplines working together is so important. The law and psychology and general medicine have to work together if we are going to create a fairer, safer and better society for everyone. Whether they have a condition or not.

Conclusion:

Truth be told, I've been putting off doing this episode for a while because I wasn't sure if I could create a long enough episode from it. But now I have I'm extremely glad because it was great to see how dementia can interact with our behaviour to cause criminality.

And this is what I love about focusing on a topic because you get to see all the little nuances, and how it impacts from different fields of psychology!

HOW TO MANAGE INCONTINENCE IN DEMENTIA?

Whilst I fully admit the next chapter of the book isn't exactly the most glamorous of topics, it is still a critical behaviour that not only occurs in the vast majority of dementia patients, but it is common in old age anyway. As well as I found it rather surprising how much information there is on incontinence, and why it is important to know about.

And one reason why it is important to know about is because whilst incontinence is not as problematic as the anger, agitation or aggression that occurs within dementia patients. Incontinence is still very upsetting for not only the person who urinates or soils themselves, but it is upsetting for the friends and family members around them. Mainly because they're the people who has to clean it up and it is still sad to see your family member go through this deterioration. As well as this is a major reason why dementia sufferers end up going into a care facility and leave home.

What Are The Types of Incontinence?

Additionally, sometimes I was a little surprised by was all the different types of incontinence that can a person can have. Since I fully believed that incontinence was only caused by weakening bladder muscles, but that's only one type.

Instead there are many different types. For example, some types are related to anatomical and medical causes, with these types best evaluated and treated by a urologist or other doctor. And if you or another you know are showing signs of this then it is important to discuss this issue with your doctor so you can get treated.

Then again the medication prescribed for this sort of thing can make thinking and memory worse.

The second type of incontinence is when a person experiences leakage when they sneeze, laugh or cough. This is known as stress incontinence with it being more common in older women and results from weakening or damage to bladder muscles that can no longer hold urine in.

Thirdly, you can have overflow incontinence occurs when the bladder doesn't completely empty, and this is common in men with enlarged prostates, but it can occur in women as well.

Penultimately, there is a type of incontinence that anyone can get, and this is known as Bowel incontinence. And the reason why this can happen to anyone is because it occurs because of problems anyone can get, like diarrhoea. It is common in dementia in the moderate and several stages for the same reasons why urinary incontinence is common.

Finally, a person can have Urge incontinence (also known as overactive bladder). This is when a person has a sudden, strong urge to urinate, and they need to run to the bathroom and they sadly don't make it there in time. Resulting in the urination or soiling themselves.

Although, some people do have milder forms of this type of incontinence, leading them to needing urge bathroom trips frequently without having incontinence itself.

What Can Make Incontinence Worse With Dementia?

Furthermore, in dementia, there are 4 things that can cause or make incontinence worse for a sufferer.

Firstly, as we know from other chapters, dementia causes a person's frontal lobes and white matter connections to become damaged so their ability to control their bladder is impaired. Resulting in them being less able to hold urine in regardless of how hard they try.

Secondly, due to the memory problems dementia causes, the person might forget to have a toilet before they go on a long walk or car ride, or just forget to adjust their fluid intakes.

Thirdly, as dementia attends to effective older people, at this age mobility can sometimes be a problem too. Therefore, if a dementia sufferer cannot move fast enough to get to the bathroom in time, they simply… you get the idea.

Finally, and this is a tragic effect of dementia, it is that some dementia sufferers simply aren't bothered if they urinate or soil themselves. As well as it's the lack of concern for basic hygiene that can be seen in the early stages of those with a frontal lobe dysfunction. Such as people with frontotemporal dementia or in the severe stage of any dementia.

Therefore, whilst this wasn't one of the pretty chapters, I think we can agree that it's important to be aware of. Especially with incontinence being an unfortunate indicator of dementia.

TREMORS IN DEMENTIA

Sort of keeping up here with the unofficial theme of this section of the book, I wanted us to look at another slightly strange and under-investigated area of dementia. And that is to do with tremors.

Since if we go back to the example of my Great-Uncle, he had really bad tremors because of his dementia and it made certain tasks next to impossible like drinking a mug of tea or coffee. The mug could end up shaking so much you always had to have a tissue or tea towel close by to mop up what was spilled.

Therefore, tremors in dementia and in elderly age are very difficult to deal with for the sufferers because they can end up making the most basic of tasks, including eating, a lot more difficult.

In addition, there are a lot of different types of tremors in dementia sufferers. As well as this is also common in people who don't suffer from dementia and a neurologist can help you or your loved one understand which type of tremor it is, with this being important because the type could be a sign of dementia or not.

Another reason why it could be important to know the sort of tremor a person is experiencing is because some tremors are down to the side effects of medication, others can be treated with specific medications, so it's important to sort out which type it is.

For example the people who unfortunately suffer with dementia with Lewy Bodies and Parkinson's disease, they have a tremor type that is generally described as "pill rolling". This is when their thumb and forefinger may move rhythmically back and forth as if person rolling a pill or pea in their hand, as well as this is sometimes seen in vascular dementia.

A second type of tremor is what's known as Enhanced Physiologic Tremor. This is normal for people to have this tremor when they're nervous or carrying something heavy, for instance. And a good way to think about this sort of tremor is it is a normal tremor that is amplified by something, with the most probable most common cause being caffeine, but prescription medication can cause it too.

Finally, the most common tremor, but one that isn't really associated with dementia or other conditions, is an "essential tremor", with this causing shaking when doing things. Like carrying a glass of water as well as this was something that the actress Katherine Hepburn developed in her later years and it runs in families.

Now this is really interesting and rather concerning because this runs in my family funnily-enough. Since I remember stories about my grandad taking the mic out of his nan for shaking so badly when she carried drinks into them, that they always wondered if they would have any tea left by the time they got the mugs.

He has the same thing now, so hopefully but I doubt it, me and my father won't get it.

Anyway, moving onto a conclusion of sorts, so we know that tremors in old age and elderly people can be very annoying and make even the most basic jobs more difficult.

To solve these tremors, medication could be tried but it rarely eliminates tremors completely.

Also if you or your loved ones have tremors and you want to help them. The problem is that people with tremors experience more difficulties using light objects like a paper cup. Therefore, it might be a good idea to use heavier items. Like heavy mugs, glasses and cutlery when drinking and eating. Due to weighted items tend to dampen effects of the tremor, making it easier to eat and drink, and thankfully these generally easy to find with you only needing to type in keywords like *weighted silverware* into the internet to get what you're looking for.

ARE DEMENTIA RATES DECLINING?

Before we move onto the last two chapters of the book, I wanted us to look at a very interesting argument and some findings from a recent study on dementia rates. The main reason why I wanted us to look at this is simply because in psychology and science as a whole, we always need to look at both sides of an argument, and dementia is no different.

Therefore, one of the subtle arguments throughout the book and in the dementia literature is that dementia rates will only grow and grow and grow over the next few decades, but this might not be the case possibly after all.

Yet if it does than all these dementia cases will put an immense pressure on our society, medical services and other public services and these will only cost more and more to taxpayers. Then there's the personal costs because families will be devastated that this is happening to their loved one and they will somehow have to pay for care.

As well as with a lot of western countries like the United Kingdom and Italy have ageing populations, these only encourage the rates of dementia cases to rise.

As a result, in an article by The Alzheimer Cohorts Consortium, they suggest that the dementia case burden might not be as bad as feared. Due to they presents results of a comprehensive research project examining thousands of people aged over 65 between 1988 and 2015.

For their study they used 9 cohort studies in United States, Sweden, the Netherlands, United Kingdom, Iceland and France, along with data collected from 49,202 participants and it must be noted that 59% of the participants were female. But as you'll see in our final chapter is this is probably not a population or sample bias, it might be a great realistic look at the dementia population.

Out of all these people studied in the cohort studies, 4,253 participants unfortunately developed some form of dementia by 2015 and the incidence of new dementia diagnosis is steadily increasing with age.

Although, against the expectations of the researchers, there was a 13% decrease in all-cause dementia per decade since 1998 with a similar decrease found for cases of Alzheimer's disease alone, as well as men showed a much higher decrease than women of 24% compared to 8%.

I know that was a lot of information in that paragraph but it's basically saying there was a lot of decreases in different groups, suggesting an overall decrease in dementia cases.

Consequently, if these trends continue in Europe and North America over the next few decades, there could be 15 million fewer dementia cases than expected in high-income countries alone.

Possibly meaning by 2040, there could be 60 million fewer new cases of dementia. That would be brilliant.

In addition, whilst this study seems to contradict earlier studies, thankfully these trends do seem fairly robust over time and across different countries.

Personally, this is a great study to look at because its methodology does use a lot of my favourite research techniques, and that's actually what makes it a very powerful study.

Since the study uses data from a lot of people and 6 different countries on two different continents. Therefore, it is a lot more difficult for critics to condemn the study for making grand conclusions based on tiny amounts of data from a single country.

Instead because there are so many participants from so many different countries and continents, these results suggest there is a universal behavioural trend going on that dementia rates are decreasing in higher income countries.

Of course, as psychology students and professionals, we always need to be balanced. So I will add that these results (like the research says) can only apply to higher income countries because no middle or lower income countries were used in the research sample, and as you'll see in the next two chapters those types of countries have their own problems.

Also, I am slightly concerned about the size of the research sample overall compared to the population of those countries. For example, off the top of my head, the USA's population is around 350 million people and according to Statista.com in 2020 16.9% of the US's population was aged over 65 giving us around 59 million people.

Therefore, even if all 49,000 participants where from the US then this isn't a very large sample and probably representative of the overall over 65 population in each country. Especially when you have stark regional differences like the USA (next chapter).

I know it's a bit picky but there are just some limitations of the research.

Possible Explanations

Building upon these findings, there are no easy explanations for why this decrease seems to be happening, but it is important to find out why says the lead author of the research Albert Hofman. As well as he acknowledges the true explanation is likely related to overall improvements in medical care over decades for older adults in high income countries.

For example, over the past few decades there have been improvements in cardiovascular treatment like statins and other medications to control blood pressure, inflammation and cholesterol, and as we saw from a previous chapter, maintaining good cardiovascular health is important to protect your health and reduce risk of dementia.

In addition, over the past few decades as the public and society as a whole have become more aware of healthy living. There have been a lot of people introducing other healthy lifestyle changes and more to help them ensure they have a healthier life, and this helps many people who might have developed dementia otherwise.

On the other hand, there has been a sharp rise in diabetes and obesity in western countries and according to Hofman (and I highly doubt any medical professional would disagree) these are two risk factors not helpful in curbing dementia.

Moreover, over the past few decades, there has been an amazing rise in access to education and other mental stimulation to older people. Like the rise in websites, online courses and other educational content.

For example, I would personally like to add that the rise of the internet has allowed older adults and everyone to access more information so they can learn and keep their minds active. As well as the rise of podcasts, like my one The Psychology World Podcast, have allowed older people to learn on the go and just listen if reading is a bit harder than it used to be.

In fact, I get a good amount of emails a year and I'm really pleased that I'm able to help these older adults learn, stay active and hopefully reduce their risk of dementia. And the same goes for eBook or print books really, they are easier and cheaper to get now so this gives older people even more access to information.

<u>Mini-Conclusion</u>

Overall, this study might be very promising and it is truly amazing that we have such a hopeful finding from research. But we cannot stop worrying about the dramatic rises in dementia cases and potential impacts, because even if the predictions are not as bad as we feared, there will still be a lot of cases that will seriously strain our loved ones and our healthcare infrastructure.

Then again, this does suggest that having proper healthcare and staying both mentally and physically active could help older adults live much longer and more productive lives.

And that's something all of us definitely want for ourselves, our friends and our loved ones.

HEALTH INEQUALITIES IN DEMENTIA HEALTHCARE

As we move towards the end of the book I wanted to address something that is absolutely critical moving forward in terms of dementia treatment and research. We need to tackle the very stark and concerning findings that massive health inequalities exist in our society and they very much affect dementia.

We're seen this clear as day over the past two years when I've writing this, due to the COVID-19 pandemic showed how ethnic minorities were not as able as their white counterparts to get access to good medical treatment, they were more likely to die from COVID-19 amongst other factors.

As well as the Black Lives Matter movement also helped to start the conversations about health inequalities in the world.

And let me be very clear here because me and other professionals wholeheartedly believe that healthcare should be accessible to every single person and treatment should be equal to everyone. Regardless of their race, gender, socioeconomic status, and all of the other silly reasons that humans discriminate against each other. Like sexual orientation.

Furthermore, especially in the United States, there is a lot of research into it (which is mentioned in the reference section at the end of the book), but research shows that wealth determines health outcomes more than genetics. That's just headshaking.

Moreover, Latinos are 1.5 times more likely to develop Alzheimer's compared to white Americans. As well as older African Americans are about twice as likely to have Alzheimer's and related dementias compared to older white Americans.

As you can see, and if you did some extra research on the internet, the effect of health inequalities is very real, and very harmful.

Personally, I think of some of the arguments racists come up with are funny about why white and other so-called "supreme" beings (what utter rubbish) need to make not blacks and other people don't get equal medical treatment. I think the funniest one was something about the blacks will end up hogging all the supplies for themselves.

It's absolutely rubbish because every good person (which the world overwhelmingly is) will share the resources with each other.

And as you'll see throughout this chapter, it is the bias and other concerns that are baked into the research and healthcare system that is causing a lot of problems for minority groups.

That's what this chapter and a lot of other people hope to address.

In addition, I'll be quoting a few times from an organisation known as UsAgainstAlzheimer's, which is an organisation that hopes to raise awareness on this issue and help tackle dementia for everyone.

Therefore, I wanted to start off with this quote:

"Stigmas, misunderstandings, and weak linkages to our nation's healthcare system are leading to significant disparities in Alzheimer's and dementia diagnosis rates, access to treatment, quality of care, and clinical research and trial participation rates among Latinos and African Americans," according to UsAgainstAlzheimer's.

Also, it's important to note that UsAgainstAlzhemier's predicts that by 2030 African Americans and Latinos will make up nearly 40% of all the 8.4 million American families affected by Alzheimer's.

For starters, it's terrible that the number will reach 8.4 million families but it is flat out terrible that a minority group that makes up 13.4% of the US population (as you'll see later) makes up a disproportionate amount of cases.

As a result, whilst the full extent of this disproportionate impact is still being studied. There are dementia risk factors, like diabetes and hypertensions, that are higher in communities of colour. Resulting in an increased risk of dementia as well.

Nevertheless, as I've hopefully showed you throughout the book, whilst some risk factors for dementia cannot change, like ageing and genetics. It is a massive misconception that dementia cannot be prevented. Since studies (references at the end of the book) have showed a third of global dementia cases can be prevented if we change some lifestyle factors. Like healthy eating, exercising regularly and getting enough sleep.

Of course, these are ideal and they sound very easy to change, but the reality is not everyone has access to the resources to make these changes.

"We are learning more and more about the interconnections between Alzheimer's risk and the social determinants of health like environmental exposures and access to healthy food. And critically, we know that racial discrimination shapes one's access to the healthcare system and to research opportunities, placing people of color at a much greater disadvantage in combating Alzheimer's through early detection, preventative health measures, and research participation," said Resendez. *"For these reasons, health equity must be a priority in our response to Alzheimer's at the community level and nationally."*

Leading us onto our next topic.

Social Determinants Of Healthcare

Our next section is about how social factors. Like our living conditions, society and environment interact and ultimately determine the healthcare we receive. For example, living in a richer area and being richer ourselves means we have better access to good medical facilities compared to poorer people in poorer neighbourhoods.

For example, a study from JAMA Neurology showed dementia is more prevalent (more common) and occurs 10 years earlier in low and middle income countries than in higher income countries. As a result of barriers, like:

- Stress
- Poor living conditions
- Poor nutrition and lack of access to healthy food (living in the food desert)
- Lack of access to education and leisure activities

This all contributes to cognitive decline.

And I actually want to highlight the lack of access to education here, because people from poorer backgrounds and neighbourhoods tend to have poorer quality of schools in their area. Resulting in them not able to get the high quality education that they need to learn about certain things.

For example, take yourself as a reader, you might only know about dementia because you're reading this book or you knew about it before and wanted to broaden your knowledge. This book in electronic format will probably retail for about $4.99 with the paperback being at least $8.99 when they both come out.

And this is a perfect example of education

inequalities to some extent. Since if you're from a poor family and need every penny or cent you can to make ends-meet then $4.99 is not a good price for you because it's probably too expensive. But if you're from a wealthier, middle class family then $5 might not be an issue for you in the slightest.

Meaning the richer reader from a middle-class family could get the very informative and engaging book about dementia and learn how to prevent it in themselves and others, for example. Whilst the poorer reader couldn't.

I know it was a quick example but it still illustrates the point about health inequalities, people without a lack of good education and prosperous backgrounds, and dementia.

Importance Of Access to Healthy Food

Another critical determinant of brain health and your own personal risk to dementia is your healthy diet as we've learnt throughout the book. Due to having access to healthy food for a healthy and balanced diet is absolutely critical to brain health.

However, I'm sure everyone is already at least somewhat familiar with this finding, but fresh fruits as well as vegetables can be cost prohibitive and result in the consumption of processed foods. Which are high in sugar and saturated fats, as well as they are cheaper to buy.

Leading poorer people to eat worst food that ends up harming their brain health in the long term.

Also if you doubt this at all, go into your local

supermarket and compare the prices of fresh fruit and vegetables to something unhealthy and processed. For example, I did this recently and even if the cheapest supermarket around, vegetables were about 60p and biscuits, small cakes and more were cheaper at something around 40p.

This is far from good for helping poorer people eat more healthily.

Additionally, according to the U.S Department of Agriculture, there are more than 23.5 million people in the United States living in food desert areas where they don't have access to supermarkets or other stores selling a variety of affordable healthy food options.

Furthermore, Vemuri et al. (2014) showed people having a lower education level is associated with higher risk of dementia and earlier symptom onset by up to eight years.

As well as stress is another risk factor for dementia and living conditions have all been associated with a higher risk of cognitive impairment, with examples of these living conditions including poverty, sexual and domestic violence and displacement.

Overall, as I'll explain more in the final chapter, it is extremely clear and concerning that your health is definitely not isolated in your biology, and that it can and is affected by a lot of non-biological factors.

That's why tackling poverty and other social determinants of healthcare is so important.

Economic Impact

Another facet, if you will, of the social determinants of healthcare is the economy and basically how much money you make and is available to you. Yet in this example, I want to highlight what dementia costs an economy.

Therefore, in the United States, there are 5 million Americans living with Alzheimer's and this number is expected to increase to 14 million in 2050, and there is no cure for dementia at this current moment in time unfortunately.

This number is just staggering considering there will be a higher prevalence rate of Alzheimer's and related dementias (ADRD) in minority groups, as supported by the following quote by Stephanie Monroe, Director of Equity and Access at UsAgainstAlzheimer's and Executive Director at AfricanAmericansAgainstAlzheimer's.

"Though blacks comprise approximately 13.4 percent of the U.S. population, we are bearing over 33 percent of the national costs of Alzheimer's,"

Moreover, this increase in cases will result in the accumulative economic cost being $2.3 trillion to Latino families by 2060 according to UsAgainstAlzheimer's.

That's a lot of money out of the pockets of a small percentage of the population. Personally, I think, only highlights the tragedy and the urgency for helping to dress these health inequalities.

Due to another way to look at it (and just maybe

this would persuade the people who want these inequalities to exist and become reinforced) is simply that if we tackle these health inequalities then the Latinos and other minority groups do not have to tackle this burden alone. Meaning they can reuse the money to improve their local community and their socioeconomic status so they can possibly end up being taxed more. Resulting in more money for everyone being available.

Personally I know I was just grasping at straws but the point is these need to be tackled and it is simply unacceptable that a small proportion needs to deal with such an extremely high cost.

How Do We Address In Dementia Psychology?

To address this, what the field of dementia sciences needs to do is to increase the diversity within clinical trials according to the U.S Food And Drug Administration. They need to people of colour and minority groups to take part in trials as these people will ultimately be a large percentage of users of the drug once approved.

Nevertheless, there are a lot of barriers to their inclusion according to the researcher Resendez.

As a result of many ADRD trials have very strict criteria that stops people with diabetes, hypertension and other conditions from taking part. This is a big problem because people of colour are more likely to have these excluding conditions compared to white and richer counterparts.

Another barrier is there is a lack of research

infrastructure that allows researchers to reach into underserved communities and connects to health providers serving people of colour.

And maybe this is the most concerning barrier, and something that became very clear due to the media coverage during the COVID-19 pandemic, but there is a long history of racism in clinical trials that has ended up eroding trust in research enterprises amongst black, indigenous and people of colour.

Some unfortunately famous cases include Henrietta Lacks, Havasupai tribe and the Tuskegee experiment. These are great examples of horribly unethical and improper research involving these communities. The effects of these continue to hinder progress in research even now.

On the other hand, there has thankfully been some progress since in 1993 the U.S's National Institutes of Health required federally funded clinical research to include women and minorities. Yet 27 years later the research still lacks ethnic diversity with 72% of the participants being white.

Additionally, data from the Food and Drug Administration shows African American participants increased from 5% in 2010 to 9% in 2019 and Latino participants increased from 1% in 2010 to 18% in 2019.

Then it's another positive that lots of charity and government bodies are getting involved in outreach work that is critical to recruiting, and making sure that minority groups are involved in the research process.

And most importantly the minority groups benefit from this research.

Conclusion:

To wrap up this penultimate chapter, I can thankfully say that we are moving in the right direction to eliminate these barriers to research, and get rid of these outrageous health inequalities that exist in our society.

Even more so with the research community starting to understand the importance of identifying and tearing down barriers preventing communities from achieving health equity.

But there is still a lot more to do and hopefully this will only continue as we, as a society, become more and more aware of these inequalities and want to get rid of them.

GENDER INEQUALITIES IN DEMENTIA HEALTHCARE

Moving onto our final chapter, in the last chapter we spoke about the health inequalities that minority groups faced so now I want to zero-in on gender inequality. Especially as I know most of the psychology audience is women, and I really want you to know that you aren't alone if you face discrimination and inequality.

But it is flat out outrageous and no woman, minority or anyone should face discrimination.

Also I want to say here that there is a lot of information in the chapter but the majority of the references are at the end of the book with the rest of them are in the chapter.

Therefore, there are 5 million Americans living with Alzheimer's or another form of dementia and according to the World Health Organisation, it is estimated there are 50 million people living with dementia globally.

Now this sounds bad enough but it is even worse because dementia is not an equal opportunity disease with two thirds of the sufferers are women. As well as based on the Aging, Demographics, and Memory Study, they estimated that amongst people aged 71 and older, 16% of women have Alzhimer's or another type of dementia compared to 11% of men.

Leading us to the critical question of why the disparity?

We know from previous chapters that age is the biggest known factor for dementia, and having a longer life expectancy is attributed as the main reason why women have higher rates of dementia than men.

For example, according to the World Health Organisation, "Women generally live longer than males — on average by six to eight years...and the extra years of life for women are not always lived in good health,"

However, this doesn't account for the gap in dementia rates for women, because there are other factors that play key roles in the unequal health outcomes women experience around cognitive health (and other health outcomes but that is beyond the scope of this book).

Social Determinants Of Healthcare

Just as a quick reminder from the last chapter, social determinants are social and environmental factors that impact your health and healthcare. For example, living conditions, poverty, wealth and more.

In addition, Sarah Lenz Lock who is the

executive director of the Global Council On Brain Health, believes that social determinants have a massive impact on women's brain health. As supported by the following quote:

"Women face more challenges due to lower educational levels, they have fewer economic resources, they provide more caregiving for their families and they experience more stress — and these factors can have an effect on the risk of cognitive decline,"

And normally I would dive into looking at these factors now but I'll unpack them in a moment later in the chapter.

To provide more support to this idea is Sandro Galeo, who is the Dean and a Professor at Boston University School of Public Health in a podcast interview with Smarter Healthcare.

"Social determinants are the housing we live in...whether there's gender equity, whether we are victims of violence, whether there are opportunities to actually live one's life fully. We tend to see health as something that happens in my body, in your body. And that approach results in a limiting. And in fact, we know now that the world around us matters much more to our health than does biology. The social factors matter much more than biology."

And this is something that I do want to mention quickly, I really like the idea of looking beyond the traditional medical-only belief about conditions. Since this links to the modern thinking about the biopsychosocial model because we need to start thinking a lot more about our psychological and social factors impact our health compared to only how our biology does.

If these past few chapters have taught me anything, it is how important the social factors are when it comes to the biological matter of dementia.

And if you've listened to my podcast and read my other books then you realise I really don't like the biomedical model, and lots of other professionals don't as well.

This is one of the reasons why.

<u>Challenges Faced By Women</u>

To look into these inequalities in a bit more depth we need to look at what challenges women face in the world, and a great place to start in looking at some research is in the USA's employment market.

Due to for the first time in 2019 women made up the majority of the university educated workforce, with 29.5 million working women compared to 29.3 million men in the workforce. But parity seems to end there.

As a result, there are fewer women in leadership roles with women only making up 27.6% of CEOs.

If we look at the US senate, only 26 of out 100 senators are women, as well as if we look at Fortune 500 companies, only 7.4% have a woman CEO.

Additionally, in the US Congress, women make up 23.7% of representatives at the national level. Which is very strange considering isn't there more women in the population than 23%?

And that just goes to highlight that none of these

statistics are representative of overall population and something (normally patriarchies and other factors we'll look at in a moment) is causing women to be blocked out of these roles.

Moreover, in the *2019 Women In the Workplace Report*, it found that 39% women said they do all or most of childcare and housework for their families, compared to just 11% of men.

As well as the problem here is these top jobs require a lot of long hours and most women still work the famous "double shift". Which I wasn't aware of until I researched this book with women working at a day job then doing the housework and all the childcare when they come home.

Overall, this makes it difficult for women to get support to succeed in leadership positions, and it much easier to focus on work and a career when someone else is doing all or most of the childcare and managing the day-to-day needs at home.

How These Challenges Impact Women's Cognition?

For the last section of the chapter, we need to see how these challenges faced by women affect their mental processes. For example, the Rotterdamn Study found that the risk of dementia in women was significantly increased for those with lower education, but education-level showed no significant effects on men.

Equally, Powell et al. (2020) showed that people who lived in disadvantaged areas had roughly twice the odds of having Alzheimer's related brain changes than people who live in the wealthiest neighbourhoods. Therefore, neighbourhoods of a poorer socioeconomic status are characterised by low levels of education, high use of public assistance and high unemployment, and as a result are more likely to cause dementia.

Thirdly, a study from Cadar et al. (2018) confirmed that the risk of dementia is higher for older adults with fewer economic resources (in other words poorer people) compared to wealthier peers. As well as a senior author of the study Professor Andrew Steptoe at University College London (UCL)'s Institute for Epidemiology and health says:

"Many factors could be involved. Differences in healthy lifestyle and medical risk factors are relevant. It may also be that better-off people have greater social and cultural opportunities that allow them to remain actively engaged with the world."

Finally, data from the U.S Census bureau found in 2017 the poverty rate for women that were 65 year olds and over was 10.5% and only 7.5% for men.

Overall, as we can see, there are a lot of impacts and challenges over the two past chapters that affect minority groups and women a lot when it comes to healthcare. Those that live in poverty, disadvantaged neighbourhoods amongst other factors are more likely to get dementia and suffer its devastating consequences.

That's why as a society we need to help address these issues so that everyone can ideally get the same level of healthcare, and no one is more likely to get dementia based on their sex, ethnic group or anything else that is quite frankly so petty and outrageous.

Of course, there are lots of great government and charity programmes throughout the world trying to address this and whilst some are working well, there is still an extremely clear need for us to do more.

There is still a long way to go but at least there is hope for the future.

CONCLUSION

After looking at a wide range of factors from the types of dementia to how to prevent it to additional information about dementia, I really hope that all of us have learnt something new about this awful range of conditions.

Dementia is not good to experience either as a person or as a loved one, and as global cases continue to rise and there continues to be no cure for it at this moment in time. This is what makes books like this and information about dementia even more critical.

Therefore, whilst nothing in this book has been official advice, I would unofficially recommend you really do start looking at your own lifestyle and seeing if there are any habits you could adopt to decrease your risk of dementia. If you don't get a good night sleep then maybe try and work out why that is and fix it. If you don't do a lot of exercise, then maybe exercise more, and if you don't eat a balanced diet, try to fix your diet.

There are so many great easy ways to help reduce your risk of getting dementia and preventing yourself for your loved ones going through so much emotional pain. You just need to find the courage to try it, and believe me I know it does take courage.

In addition, this is also important information to spread and try to help make other people aware. So please, share this book with friends, family and other loved ones so they can become aware of dementia, its risk and how to reduce it.

The entire purpose of this book has been to help people so they hopefully don't have to go through what my family did over the past few years, I don't wish that on anyone.

So I hoped you enjoyed the book and learnt something. If you did then that is a total win in my opinion. Have a great day and hopefully I'll see you in another book soon.

REFERENCE LIST

Budson AE, O'Connor MK. Seven Steps to Managing Your Memory: What's Normal, What's Not, and What to Do About It, New York: Oxford University Press, 2017.

Budson AE, Solomon PR. Memory Loss, Alzheimer's Disease, & Dementia: A Practical Guide for Clinicians, 2nd Edition, Philadelphia: Elsevier Inc., 2016.

Liljegren, M., Naasan, G., Temlett, J., Perry, D. C., Rankin, K. P., Merrilees, J., Grinberg, L. T., Seeley, W. W., Englund, E., & Miller, B. L. (2015). Criminal behavior in frontotemporal dementia and Alzheimer's disease. *JAMA neurology*, *72*(3), 295–300. https://doi.org/10.1001/jamaneurol.2014.3781

About Racial and Ethnic Disparities in Alzheimer's. (n.d.). UsAgainstAlzheimer's. Retrieved from https://www.usagainstalzheimers.org/learn/disparities

Resende EDPF, Llibre Guerra JJ, Miller BL. Health and

Socioeconomic Inequities as Contributors to Brain Health. JAMA Neurol. 2019;76(6):633–634. doi:10.1001/jamaneurol.2019.0362

African Americans and Alzheimer's Disease: The Silent Epidemic. (n.d.). Alzheimer's Association. Retrieved from https://www.alz.org/media/Documents/african-americans-silent-epidemic-r.pdf

Allen, K. (2018, Sept 27). Dementia Cases to Grow Substantially Among African Americans, Hispanics. AARP. Retrieved from https://www.aarp.org/health/dementia/info-2018/dementia-alzheimer-cases-grow-nonwhites.html

Monroe, S., Resendez, J. (2019, April 30). Addressing Injustice in Alzheimer's and Bringing Brain Health Equity to Communities of Color. UsAgainstAlzheimer's. Retrieved from https://www.usagainstalzheimers.org/blog/addressing-injustice-alzheimers-and-bringing-brain-health-equity-communities-color

Livingston, G., Sommerlad, A., Orgeta, V., Costafreda, S. G., Huntley, J., Ames, D., ... & Cooper, C. (2017). Dementia prevention, intervention, and care. The Lancet, 390(10113), 2673-2734. https://www.thelancet.com/journals/lancet/article/PIIS0140-6736(17)31363-6/fulltext#seccestitle70

Yaffe K, Vittinghoff E, Lindquist K, et al. Posttraumatic stress disorder and risk of dementia among US veterans. Arch Gen Psychiatry. 2010;67 (6):608-613. doi:10.1001/archgenpsychiatry. 2010.61

Ver Ploeg M. Access to affordable, nutritious food is limited in "food deserts." United States Department of Agriculture. Updated March 1, 2010.

Social Determinants of Health. (n.d.). Office of Disease Prevention and Health Promotion. Retrieved from https://www.healthypeople.gov/2020/topics-objectives/topic/social-determinants-of-health

2019 Drug Trials Snapshots Summary Report (n.d.). U.S. Food and Drug Administration. Retrieved from https://www.fda.gov/media/135337/download

Racial and Ethnic Disparities in Alzheimer's Disease: A Literature Review. (2014, February 1). Office of the Assistant Secretary for Planning and Evaluation. Retrieved from https://aspe.hhs.gov/report/racial-and-ethnic-disparities-alzheimers-disease-literature-review

Together We Success: Accelerating Research on Alzheimer's Disease and Related Dementias (n.d.) National Institutes of Health. Retrieved from https://www.nia.nih.gov/sites/default/files/2019-07/FY21-bypass-budget-report-508.pdf

Hendrie HC, Smith-Gamble V, Lane KA, Purnell C, Clark DO, Gao S. The Association of Early Life Factors and Declining Incidence Rates of Dementia in an Elderly Population of African Americans. J Gerontol B Psychol Sci Soc Sci. 2018;73(suppl_1):S82-S89. doi:10.1093/geronb/gbx143

Diversity in Clinical Trials. (n.d.). Clinical Research Pathways. Retrieved from https://clinicalresearchpathways.org/diversity/

Twenty-seven-year time trends in dementia incidence in Europe and the United States. The Alzheimer Cohorts Consortium, Frank J. Wolters, Lori B. Chibnik, et al Neurology Aug 2020, 95 (5) e519-e531; (Open Acccess)

Budson AE, Solomon PR. Memory Loss, Alzheimer's Disease, & Dementia: A Practical Guide for Clinicians, 3rd Edition, Philadelphia: Elsevier Inc., 2021.

Quantifying America's Gender Wage Gap by Race/Ethnicity. (2020, March). National Partnership for Women and Families. Retrieved from https://www.nationalpartnership.org/our-work/resources/economic-justice/fair-pay/quantifying-americas-gender-wage-gap.pdf

Michals, D. (Ed.) (2017). Lucretia Mott. (n.d.). National Women's History Museum. Retrieved from https://www.womenshistory.org/education-resources/biographies/lucretia-mott

Michals, D. (Ed.) (2017). Elizabeth Cady Stanton. (n.d.) National Women's History Museum. Retrieved from https://www.womenshistory.org/education-resources/biographies/elizabeth-cady-stanton

Hayward, N. (Ed) (2018). Susan B. Anthony. (n.d.) National Women's History Museum. Retrieved from https://www.womenshistory.org/education-resources/biographies/susan-b-anthony

Norwood, A. (2017). Ida B. Wells-Barnett. National Women's History Museum. Retrieved from https://www.womenshistory.org/education-resources/biographies/ida-b-wells-barnett

Alexander, K. (2018-2020). Frances Ellen Watkins Harper. National Women's History Museum. Retrieved from https://www.womenshistory.org/education-resources/biographies/frances-ellen-watkins-harper

19th Amendment. (2020, August 14). History.com. Retrieved from https://www.history.com/topics/womens-history/19th-amendment-1

Facts and Figures. (n.d.). Alzheimer's Association. Retrieved from https://www.alz.org/alzheimers-dementia/facts-figures

10 Facts on Dementia. (2019, September). World Health Organization. Retrieved from https://www.who.int/features/factfiles/dementia/en/

Plassman, B. L., Langa, K. M., Fisher, G. G., Heeringa, S. G., Weir, D. R., Ofstedal, M. B., Burke, J. R., Hurd, M. D., Potter, G. G., Rodgers, W. L., Steffens, D. C., Willis, R. J., & Wallace, R. B. (2007). Prevalence of dementia in the United States: the aging, demographics, and memory study. Neuroepidemiology, 29(1-2), 125–132. https://doi.org/10.1159/000109998

Female life expectancy. (n.d.). World Health Organization. Retrieved from https://www.who.int/gho/women_and_health/mortality/situation_trends_life_expectancy/en/

About Alzheimer's. (n.d.). Women's Alzheimer's

Movement. Retrieved from https://thewomensalzheimersmovement.org/about-alzheimers/

Colino, S. (2020, May 20). Dementia's Gender Disparity: Report Uncovers Unique Challenges Facing Women. AARP. Retrieved from https://www.aarp.org/health/brain-health/info-2020/dementia-women-risk-caregiving.html

Fry, R. (2019, June 20). U.S. women near milestone in the college-educated labor force. Pew Research Center. Retrieved from https://www.pewresearch.org/fact-tank/2019/06/20/u-s-women-near-milestone-in-the-college-educated-labor-force/?

Livingston, G., Huntley, J., Sommerlad, A., Ames, D., Ballard, C., Banerjee, S., Brayne, C., Burns, A., Cohen-Mansfield, J., Cooper, C., Costafreda, S. G., Dias, A., Fox, N., Gitlin, L. N., Howard, R., Kales, H. C., Kivimäki, M., Larson, E. B., Ogunniyi, A., Orgeta, V., … Mukadam, N. (2020). Dementia prevention, intervention, and care: 2020 report of the Lancet Commission. Lancet (London, England), 396(10248), 413–446. https://doi.org/10.1016/S0140-6736(20)30367-6

Women in the Workplace 2019. (2019). Lean in & McKinsey and Company. Retrieved from https://wiw-report.s3.amazonaws.com/Women_in_the_Workplace_2019.pdf

A. Ott, C.T. M. van Rossum, F. van Harskamp, H. van de Mheen, A. Hofman, M.M. B. Breteler (1999). Education and the incidence of dementia in a large population-based study: The Rotterdam Study. Neurology. 52 (3) 663; https://doi.org/10.1212/WNL.52.3.663

Powell, WR., Buckingham, WR., Larson, JL., et al. (2020) Association of Neighborhood-Level Disadvantage With Alzheimer Disease Neuropathology. JAMA Netw Open.3(6):e207559. https://doi.org/10.1001/jamapsychiatry.2018.1012

Cadar, D., Lassale, C., Davies, H., Llewellyn, DJ., Batty, GD., Steptoe, A. (2018). Individual and Area-Based Socioeconomic Factors Associated With Dementia Incidence in England: Evidence From a 12-Year Follow-up in the English Longitudinal Study of Ageing. JAMA Psychiatry. 75(7):723–732. https://doi.org/10.1001/jamapsychiatry.2018.1012

Current Population Survey, 2018 Annual Social and Economic Supplement. U.S. Census Bureau. Retrieved from https://www.census.gov/content/dam/Census/library/visualizations/2018/demo/p60-263/figure5.pdf

Underpaid and overloaded: women in low-wage jobs. (2014). National Women's Law Center. Retrieved from https://nwlc.org/wp-content/uploads/2015/08/final_nwlc_lowwagerepor

t2014.pdf

WomenAgainstAlzheimer's. (n.d.). UsAgainstAlzheimer's. Retrieved from https://www.usagainstalzheimers.org/networks/women

Galea, S., Tracy, M., Hoggatt, K. J., Dimaggio, C., & Karpati, A. (2011). Estimated deaths attributable to social factors in the United States. American journal of public health, 101(8), 1456–1465. https://doi.org/10.2105/AJPH.2010.300086

Covinsky, K.E., Newcomer, R., Dane, C.K., Sands, L.P., Yaffe, K. (2003). Patient and caregiver characteristics associated with depression in caregivers of patients with dementia. Journal of General Internal Medicine, 18: 1006-14.

Alzheimer's Association & National Alliance for Caregiving. (2004). Families Care: Alzheimer's Caregiving in the United States. Chicago, IL: Alzheimer's Association and Bethesda, MD: National Alliance for Caregiving.

Labor Force Statistics from the Current Population Survey. (2019). U.S. Bureau of Labor Statistics. Retrieved from https://www.bls.gov/cps/cpsaat11.htm

Sucich, K. (Host). (2020, July 2). Social determinants of health, COVID-19, and racism in healthcare [Audio Podcast]. Retrieved from https://www.smarthcpodcast.com/episodes/s1-e8-sandro-galea

Hinchcliffe, E. (2020, May 18). Women run 37 Fortune

500 Companies, a record high. Fortune. Retrieved from https://fortune.com/2020/05/18/women-run-37-fortune-500-companies-a-record-high/

Women Senators. (n.d.). United States Senate. Retrieved from https://www.senate.gov/senators/ListofWomenSenators.htm

Women in the U.S. Congress 2020. (n.d.). Rutgers Eagleton Institute of Politics. Retrieved from https://cawp.rutgers.edu/women-us-congress-2020

Cassidy-Eagle, E.L. & Siebern, A. (2017). Sleep and mild cognitive impairment, *Sleep Science and Practice*, 1:15, DOI 10.1186/s41606-017-0016-5

Da Silva, R. A. P. C. (2015). Sleep disturbances and mild cognitive impairment: A review. *Sleep Science*, 8(1), 36–41. http://doi.org/10.1016/j.slsci.2015.02.001

Petersen, R. C., (2011). Mild Cognitive Impairment. New England Journal of Medicine, 364, p. 2227 - 2234.

Petit, D., Montplaisir, J., St. Louis, E.K., & Boeve, B.F., (2017). Alzheimer Disease and Other Dementias, in Kryger, M., Roth, T., Dement, W.C. (Eds.), (2017). *Principles and Practice of Sleep Medicine Sixth Edition*, Philadelphia, PA: Elsevier.

https://www.statista.com/statistics/457822/share-of-old-age-population-in-the-total-us-population/

Alzheimer's Research UK- https://www.alzheimersresearchuk.org/wp-content/uploads/2021/04/YourBrainMatters_Apr2021.pdf

Graff-Radford, J. & Lunde, A. M. (2020). *Mayo Clinic on Alzheimer's Disease and Other Dementias*. Rochester, MN: Mayo Clinic Press, pp. 48 ff, p. 290-1.

Sing out. "Choir Singing Can Improve Cognitive Functioning Among the Elderly." ScienceDaily, 2.10.2021.

Sauna bathing. Emamzadeh, A. "Could Sauna Bathing Have Cognitive Benefits?" 2.6.2021. Psychologytoday.com.

Tai chi. Harvard Health Letter of 8.22.2019.

Attitudes/Becca Levy. Applewhite, A. *This Chair Rocks: A Manifesto Against Ageism* (2016). NY: Celadon Books. pp. 43, 114

Vaccination. "Flu, pneumonia vaccinations tied to lower risk of Alzheimer's dementia." ScienceDaily, 27 July 2020.

Positive outlook. "Positive Outlook Predicts Less Memory Decline," Association for Psychology Science, 10/29/2020.

Berries, apples, green tea. "More berries, apples and tea may have protective benefits against Alzheimer's," ScienceDaily, May 5, 2020.

Coffee and dementia risk. Hendrick, B. "Coffee Strong Enough to Ward Off Dementia?" WebMd, Jan. 16, 2009.

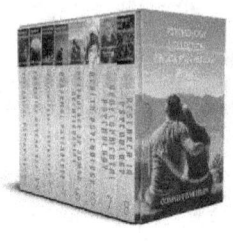
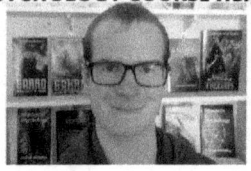

https://www.subscribepage.com/psychologyboxset

CHECK OUT THE PSYCHOLOGY WORLD PODCAST FOR MORE PSYCHOLOGY INFORMATION! AVAILABLE ON ALL MAJOR PODCAST APPS.

About the author:

Connor Whiteley is the author of over 60 books in the sci-fi fantasy, nonfiction psychology and books for writer's genre and he is a Human Branding Speaker and Consultant.

He is a passionate warhammer 40,000 reader, psychology student and author.

Who narrates his own audiobooks and he hosts The Psychology World Podcast.

All whilst studying Psychology at the University of Kent, England.

Also, he was a former Explorer Scout where he gave a speech to the Maltese President in August 2018 and he attended Prince Charles' 70th Birthday Party at Buckingham Palace in May 2018.

Plus, he is a self-confessed coffee lover!

All books in 'An Introductory Series':
Careers In Psychology
Psychology of Suicide
Dementia Psychology
Forensic Psychology of Terrorism And Hostage-Taking
Forensic Psychology of False Allegations
Year In Psychology
BIOLOGICAL PSYCHOLOGY 3RD EDITION
COGNITIVE PSYCHOLOGY THIRD EDITION
SOCIAL PSYCHOLOGY- 3RD EDITION
ABNORMAL PSYCHOLOGY 3RD EDITION
PSYCHOLOGY OF RELATIONSHIPS- 3RD EDITION
DEVELOPMENTAL PSYCHOLOGY 3RD EDITION
HEALTH PSYCHOLOGY
RESEARCH IN PSYCHOLOGY
A GUIDE TO MENTAL HEALTH AND TREATMENT AROUND THE WORLD- A GLOBAL LOOK AT DEPRESSION
FORENSIC PSYCHOLOGY
THE FORENSIC PSYCHOLOGY OF THEFT, BURGLARY AND OTHER

CRIMES AGAINST PROPERTY
CRIMINAL PROFILING: A FORENSIC PSYCHOLOGY GUIDE TO FBI PROFILING AND GEOGRAPHICAL AND STATISTICAL PROFILING.
CLINICAL PSYCHOLOGY FORMULATION IN PSYCHOTHERAPY
PERSONALITY PSYCHOLOGY AND INDIVIDUAL DIFFERENCES
CLINICAL PSYCHOLOGY REFLECTIONS VOLUME 1
CLINICAL PSYCHOLOGY REFLECTIONS VOLUME 2
Clinical Psychology Reflections Volume 3
CULT PSYCHOLOGY
Police Psychology

A Psychology Student's Guide To University
How Does University Work?
A Student's Guide To University And Learning
University Mental Health and Mindset

OTHER SHORT STORIES BY CONNOR WHITELEY

<u>Mystery Short Stories:</u>

A Smokey Way To Go

A Spicy Way To GO

A Marketing Way To Go

A Missing Way To Go

A Showering Way To Go

Poison In The Candy Cane

Christmas Innocence

You Better Watch Out

Christmas Theft

Trouble In Christmas

Smell of The Lake

Problem In A Car

Theft, Past and Team

Embezzler In The Room

A Strange Way To Go

A Horrible Way To Go

Ann Awful Way To Go

An Old Way To Go

A Fishy Way To Go

A Pointy Way To Go

A High Way To Go

A Fiery Way To Go

A Glassy Way To Go

A Chocolatey Way To Go

Kendra Detective Mystery Collection Volume 1
Kendra Detective Mystery Collection Volume 2
Stealing A Chance At Freedom
Glassblowing and Death
Theft of Independence
Cookie Thief
Marble Thief
Book Thief
Art Thief
Mated At The Morgue
The Big Five Whoopee Moments
Stealing An Election
Mystery Short Story Collection Volume 1
Mystery Short Story Collection Volume 2

Science Fiction Short Stories:
Gummy Bear Detective
The Candy Detective
What Candies Fear
The Blurred Image
Shattered Legions
The First Rememberer
Life of A Rememberer
System of Wonder
Lifesaver

Remarkable Way She Died
The Interrogation of Annabella Stormic
Blade of The Emperor
Arbiter's Truth
Computation of Battle
Old One's Wrath
Puppets and Masters
Ship of Plague
Interrogation
Edge of Failure
One Way Choice
Acceptable Losses
Balance of Power
Good Idea At The Time
Escape Plan
Escape In The Hesitation
Inspiration In Need
Singing Warriors
Knowledge is Power
Killer of Polluters
Climate of Death
The Family Mailing Affair
Defining Criminality
The Martian Affair
A Cheating Affair
The Little Café Affair
Mountain of Death

Prisoner's Fight
Claws of Death
Bitter Air
Honey Hunt
Blade On A Train

<u>Fantasy Short Stories:</u>
City of Snow
City of Light
City of Vengeance
Dragons, Goats and Kingdom
Smog The Pathetic Dragon
Don't Go In The Shed
The Tomato Saver
The Remarkable Way She Died
The Bloodied Rose
Asmodia's Wrath
Heart of A Killer
Emissary of Blood
Dragon Coins
Dragon Tea
Dragon Rider
Sacrifice of the Soul
Heart of The Flesheater
Heart of The Regent
Heart of The Standing
Feline of The Lost

Heart of The Story
City of Fire
Awaiting Death

Other books by Connor Whiteley:

Bettie English Private Eye Series

A Very Private Woman

The Russian Case

A Very Urgent Matter

A Case Most Personal

Trains, Scots and Private Eyes

The Federation Protects

The Fireheart Fantasy Series

Heart of Fire

Heart of Lies

Heart of Prophecy

Heart of Bones

Heart of Fate

City of Assassins (Urban Fantasy)

City of Death

City of Marytrs

City of Pleasure

City of Power

Agents of The Emperor

Return of The Ancient Ones

Vigilance

Angels of Fire

Kingmaker

The Eight
The Lost Generation
Lord Of War Trilogy (Agents of The Emperor)
Not Scared Of The Dark
Madness
Burn It All Down

The Garro Series- Fantasy/Sci-fi
GARRO: GALAXY'S END
GARRO: RISE OF THE ORDER
GARRO: END TIMES
GARRO: SHORT STORIES
GARRO: COLLECTION
GARRO: HERESY
GARRO: FAITHLESS
GARRO: DESTROYER OF WORLDS
GARRO: COLLECTIONS BOOK 4-6
GARRO: MISTRESS OF BLOOD
GARRO: BEACON OF HOPE
GARRO: END OF DAYS

Winter Series- Fantasy Trilogy Books
WINTER'S COMING
WINTER'S HUNT
WINTER'S REVENGE
WINTER'S DISSENSION

<u>Miscellaneous:</u>
RETURN
FREEDOM
SALVATION
Reflection of Mount Flame
The Masked One
The Great Deer

<u>Gay Romance Novellas</u>
Breaking, Nursing, Repairing A Broken Heart
Jacob And Daniel
Fallen For A Lie

www.ingramcontent.com/pod-product-compliance
Lightning Source LLC
LaVergne TN
LVHW011846060526
838200LV00054B/4190